Hannah
xx

54 Ways To Keep Your Family Healthy

Hannah Bailey

Fisher King Publishing

54 Ways To Keep Your Family Healthy

ISBN 978-1-906377-69-4

Fisher King Publishing Ltd
The Studio
Arthington Lane
Pool-in-Wharfedale
LS21 1JZ
England

This book is dedicated to my Grandpa, Eric Rowley, who is truly inspirational and has always believed in me.

I would also like to thank my family and friends for their support. Without them I would not be where I am today.

Introduction

When I graduated from Sheffield Hallam University in 2010 with a degree in Public Health Nutrition, I knew I wanted to help people understand why a healthy lifestyle is so important and how to implement that in their everyday lives.

I am passionate about healthy living and want to share with others the benefits of what I have discovered.

I see and hear so many families who struggle to eat healthily and it needn't be as difficult as some may think. There is so much advice and information out there which is wrong and causes confusion, so I wanted to put my top tips into an easy to use guide to help people make healthy choices.

Healthy eating doesn't have to be time consuming or expensive, especially if you shop locally, but it's vital for a long, healthy, happy and enjoyable life.

I hope this book will help you enjoy healthy living and reap the rewards with your family long into the future.

Break it down

If you want to improve your health, make small changes.

Trying to alter everything all at once is likely to result in you feeling overwhelmed and struggling to keep going with every change. It's at this point that you are more likely to give up and revert to old habits. View it as a long term process which needs to be taken a little piece at a time.

Pick one thing to change each week. For example, drinking a glass of water every morning when you get up or eating a piece of fruit mid-morning rather than biscuits. Small steps are more likely to lead to changes being permanent.

Remove the words 'Diet' and 'Calorie' from your mind and replace them with 'healthy lifestyle'. Ask yourself what is realistic for you and your family? What aspects do you want to improve? If you have fussy children, it may be that you want to broaden their diet. What are your personal goals? What are your partner's goals? How will you organise your meals, activities etc., around the family schedule?

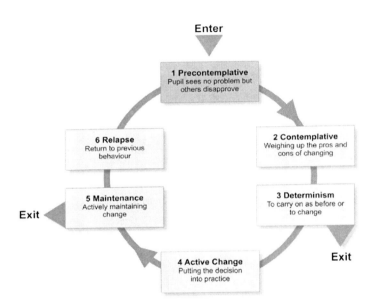

From: www.facilitatingchange.org.uk/images/model.gif

Mind over matter

When you decide to make changes to your lifestyle, mind over matter is key.

You may be aware that you need to lose weight but if you don't feel able to start making dietary changes then it becomes very difficult and de-motivating. This is when the tendency to go on a fad diet starts because they are quick fixes. Cue days of being hungry; miserable and generally fed up all in the name of losing weight. Wouldn't it be better to eat food, feel happy and not constantly hungry?

So, when you feel ready, change your mind-set to that of leading a healthy lifestyle, one step at a time. Feeling mentally ready to change is the hardest part, once you feel comfortable, putting it in to practise will come much easier.

Take a look at the diagram opposite and work out where you fit in to it. Accept you may not be at the right point to change but go back to it when you feel ready.

Relapse can happen

Any process which involves your brain and a change in behaviour always has a chance for relapse to occur, as the diagram in the previous tip shows.

Relapse happens and it is ok if it does. How you deal with it will affect what happens after that.

Don't beat yourself up and view it as failure. You have not failed; introducing negative language will make you feel more negative than you already do.

Sit down and think about how you feel. Ask yourself these questions. Be honest but fair rather than harsh:

- Why have you relapsed?
- How have you reacted?
- What happened that triggered the change in eating habits and why did you react in the way you did?
- Did you notice any warning signs that you might pick up on next time and change your reaction?

Sometimes, writing down your feelings will help you to move forward and carry on with life. This is really important. If you binged, accept it and move on. Try to go back to the good habits you had already made and view what happened as a blip.

Treat night!

Include a treat night once a week for the whole family. It might be a takeaway at the weekend, DVD and popcorn on the sofa or something nice for the children and something for you and your partner.

When depriving yourself of food you enjoy, suddenly it's everywhere and all you can think of. This generally leads you to then binge on food which kick starts the guilty feeling because you have over indulged and spoiled the 'diet'. Including a small chocolate bar a couple of times a week and not feeling the need to binge on it is far better for your physical and mental health than depriving yourself, unless you are the kind of person who prefers to go cold turkey and has to give something up completely.

This change in attitude from a diet to lifestyle choices stops the calorie, points or sins counting and allows you to enjoy food as part of a healthy balanced lifestyle. There is no need to feel guilty for the odd packet of crisps or chocolate bar through the week so long as the rest of your diet is healthy.

Diet diaries

If you are looking to lose weight, keep a diet diary. It is amazing how much extra we consume that gets forgotten about on a daily basis.

Write down all the food you eat with quantities and any that was left at the time of consumption as later recall can be poor. Also, include how much you have drunk. Each day, we consume approximately 500 calories from drinks without realising.

If you are out and about, try an app on a smart phone to help you monitor what you do. 'My fitness pal' and 'my diet diary' are apps which are highly rated but you may find a better one for you.

Alternatively, buy yourself a nice notebook and keep track of everything you eat and drink. Don't buy the cheapest one you come across, it devalues your efforts and your goals. Put your goals in the front and reflect upon them often so you can see how well you're doing with staying on track. Each week set a small goal such as not finishing everyone else's food and write this down too. Use goals to motivate you but also, accept that not meeting your goal is ok and may happen from time to time.

Watch the weighing

If you're reading this book to help you lose weight, chances are you have been weighing yourself on a regular basis in the hope that a bit more weight has come off. Weighing yourself all the time can be the start of a very slippery slope in terms of heading for an eating disorder. If you are going to use the scales to measure your weight loss, weigh yourself no more than once or twice a week.

When you're losing weight, it's not just weight that you want to see drop off but also the inches. Measure yourself once a month or once a fortnight with a tape measure to see how your body shape is changing. This is just as important as pounds off the scale. Losing weight is fine but you may be losing muscle which you don't want to do. Muscle keeps your metabolic rate higher and therefore helps with the weight loss.

Aim for 1-2lbs of weight loss each week. Depending on how much you have to lose, it may be more to begin with but if you lose too much too quickly, it won't be sustainable.

Don't put off until tomorrow that which can be done today

Although it's a bit of a cliché, it's true, even for losing weight or making lifestyle changes. Saying you will start on Monday is unlikely to ever happen as something will occur and suddenly losing weight is the last thing on your mind. Make changes slowly and gradually at a time that feels right for you and your family.

When you are looking at what you have eaten, don't view unhealthy food as failing and therefore stop bothering with trying to eat healthily. Wipe the slate clean and do something healthy such as drink a glass of water, munch on nuts or seeds and forget about the unhealthy food you ate earlier.

By putting it off until after the weekend, there is the tendency to over indulge through the weekend which makes changing more difficult as your body has a lot of sugar and other toxins or artificial products in it causing more cravings.

Make a small change today and accept that we all have a bad day once in a while but things don't have to go downhill because of it. You can get back on track.

Sleep

The average person needs around eight hours sleep. You may need eight hours of sleep! Children need more depending upon their age. Sleep is vital for the body because it's your body's chance to repair and renew itself as well as rest.

Not getting enough sleep is believed to raise the risk of many diseases in particular, stroke and obesity.

If you are looking to lose weight, having enough sleep can help curb your cravings as you don't crave sugar and caffeine as much as you do to help keep you awake. You can only survive on a few hours' sleep a night for so long before you become completely exhausted and crave carbohydrates, fizzy drinks or caffeine. If you avoid getting to this point it will help you manage your eating better which in turn impacts on your mental health.

Children also need enough sleep for the same reasons. It is widely recognised that a good bedtime routine and an undisturbed night's sleep will make for happy and healthy children.

Make sure children have enough sleep and are in bed at a suitable time especially if your child does not sleep in after a late night.

Healthy and hydrated

Drink plenty of water. There are various recommendations for how much adults should drink but aim for 1.5 to 2 litres of water a day to ensure you stay hydrated. Children's recommendations are based more on their weight but as a guide urine should be a straw colour and have no odour.

Tea, coffee and fizzy drinks do not count towards fluid intake as they contain caffeine which is a diuretic and makes you pass urine more than you would just drinking water.

Being dehydrated can have many effects. Thirst can often be confused with hunger causing us to eat more than we need. Dehydration can make you feel tired and lethargic. It can also cause headaches, dizziness and nausea. Just being dehydrated by 2% can have adverse effects on the body.

In hot weather, it is particularly important to stay well hydrated especially for young children who can become dehydrated very quickly due to their small size.

Always carry a water bottle with you and leave a glass/bottle of water on your desk to make sure you drink regularly. This will also help with concentration at work or at school for children.

Ditch the fizz

Limit fizzy drinks to a maximum of one glass a week
and encourage children to drink other liquids such as
water, squash or a glass of fruit juice once a day.

You may find it easier to go cold turkey or set
yourself a day of the week you are allowed a small
fizzy drink such as a Saturday treat. If you drink fizzy
drinks when you are out, try different fruit juices but
beware of the sugar content, try sparkling water
instead.

Although they are hugely popular especially with
teenagers, they can have serious consequences to
health which are often not realised. Not only do fizzy
drinks not quench your thirst, the full fat versions are
laden with sugar and empty calories and the diet
versions are full of artificial products of which no one
really knows the long term health consequences.

Studies have shown that drinking fizzy drinks can
cause Calcium to leach out of your bones making
them weaker, increasing the risk of osteoporosis. This
can be a particular problem in women who are
more at risk of osteoporosis than men.

Other studies have also suggested drinking diet
drinks may cause you to crave more sugary foods as
your body expects sugar but then doesn't receive
any. They are very popular with slimmers but they
could actually be making it harder to lose weight?

Cut the caffeine

Want to feel healthier and have more energy? Cut the caffeine!

Caffeine is found in a lot of common drinks such as tea, coffee, hot chocolate. Some herbal teas contain a different form of caffeine.

Most of us drink caffeine to help wake us up and then keep us going throughout the day but caffeine is seriously addictive stuff. Whilst it does wake you up, keep you awake and help you get through the day, it can also stop you sleeping at night.

Caffeine is a stimulant and therefore increases the speed of everything in your body. This is why if you drink too much, you may shake, feel anxious and have palpitations. Caffeine can also have an effect on your digestive system especially if you suffer from certain conditions such as IBS. If you notice these symptoms, try cutting down the amount of caffeine you drink and see if it improves. It can also cause mood swings in some people and the chemicals in fizzy drinks can make it even more addictive.

Try reducing your intake slowly and see how you feel. It would be good to replace caffeinated drinks with water.

Watch the fruit juices!

Whilst fruit juices and smoothies can count as 1 of your 5 a day, they are high in sugar and low in fibre so stick to one 200ml glass per day.

Fruit juices and smoothies are a great way to get some vitamins into children but make sure you check the packaging has the 1 of your 5 a day logo on otherwise they are just drinking a very sugary drink.

Due to the processing of fruit juice, much of the fibre is lost and this is one of the reasons it can only count as 1 of your 5 a day. No matter how much you drink, it only counts as 1 portion. Fruit and vegetables have a much higher fibre and lower sugar content. It is also the high sugar content and therefore higher calorie content which has caused health professionals to make this recommendation.

Don't be fooled into thinking swapping coke for fruit juice will help you lose weight because in terms of calories they are roughly the same. Replace with water for a happy, healthy, hydrated family.

Abandon the alcohol

If you want to lose weight or just be healthier, abandon the alcohol.

Alcohol has negative effects on your physical and mental health. It is a depressant and therefore despite what you may think or have been told, it won't solve your problems.

Whilst alcohol may make you feel better at the time, it is unlikely to have long term benefits. It slows down every response in the body and effectively does the opposite to caffeine. Combining the two can be dangerous.

Alcohol is also addictive and can have much more serious effects on your body if you become addicted or drink heavily regularly. Not only is alcohol full of calories with very little nutritional value, it can also damage your liver and heart and may increase the risk of some cancers namely throat, mouth and liver.

Studies suggest red wine may have positive effects on various conditions however the evidence is patchy so drink moderately.

What is moderate?

The government tell us to drink sensibly and in moderation but what does that mean when you're drinking? Men are advised to consume no more than between 3 and 4 units per night, no more than 21 in a week and have 2 alcohol free days. Women are advised to consume no more than 2-3 units per night, no more than 14 units per week and also have 2 alcohol free days. Pregnant women and women trying to conceive are advised not to drink at all.

How does that advice translate into what you're drinking?

1 unit of alcohol is equal to:

- ½ pint standard strength beer or cider (3-4%)
- A small pub measure (25ml) of spirits (40% volume)

1 ½ units of alcohol is equal to:

- A 125ml glass of wine (remember most people have larger)
- A standard pub measure (35ml) of spirits (40% volume) such as vodka

A bottle of wine has on average 9 units which is more than double the recommendations for men and women. Think about how much you drink and the risks you are posing to your health. Try to cut down by 1 glass each time you drink and reduce the frequency to avoid becoming alcohol dependant.

Start the day the healthy way

Breakfast is the most important meal of the day. Don't let anyone leave home without it! Breakfast literally breaks the fast between the last time you ate and the point at which you have breakfast. Eating it speeds up your metabolism which your body has slowed down during the night meaning you start burning calories again which, if you are looking to lose weight, is an important factor.

Studies show eating breakfast improves concentration in both adults and children. If you want your child to do well at school, they need a healthy breakfast. Most cereals are packed full of sugar and salt which are not good for us. They also are often not very filling and have a bigger impact on blood sugar so why not try these options which will keep you going longer and release energy more slowly.

- Baked beans on wholemeal toast
- Egg on wholemeal toast
- Porridge with chopped fruit
- Scrambled egg with bacon and baked beans or grilled tomatoes
- Weetabix with chopped banana

Make sure you have a glass of water too before you leave the house.

Sneaky snacks

Sack the snacks! Unless you snack on fruit, vegetables, nuts or seeds, you need to get rid of them all! Cakes, biscuits, cereal bars, crisps etc., are all full of rubbish and probably the reason you feel rubbish most of the time too.

Replace your usual snacks with the healthy ones and get rid of the unhealthy ones. Snacking on sugary foods will send your blood sugar high which in turn causes it to fall rapidly. This is what usually causes the mid-morning and mid-afternoon energy slumps we experience after having a high GI breakfast and lunch.

If you want to keep your blood sugar stable and prevent those cravings between meals, eating vegetable sticks and a small amount of dip, nuts or seeds is the best option. Some fruit contains more sugar than others especially dried fruit. That's not to say you shouldn't eat it but you may notice it making you crave sugar. Also, beware of the sugar which is often added to dried fruit. It does however, make a great portable snack if you are on the move a lot and find fruit tends to get squashed. Combine with nuts and seeds for a healthy snack.

Cubes of cheese and full fat yoghurt make great snacks for children who need a slightly lower fibre and higher fat diet than us due to their growth.

Nutty about nuts

I mentioned nuts in my last tip so why are they so good for us?

Nuts such as cashews (unsalted), walnuts and almonds have been linked to lowering cholesterol which is believed to be a cause of heart attacks and strokes, better weight control and possibly reducing the risk of certain cancers.

Walnuts are the richest source of omega 3 compared to other nuts. Omega 3 fatty acids help fight inflammation. They are also a great source of omega 3 for those that don't like or don't eat fish. As well as containing omega 3, walnuts also contain a high level of antioxidants which help prevent cancer because they scavenge free radicals which may cause cancer.

Nuts are also high in fibre which can help prevent constipation and keep you feeling fuller for longer. Almonds are especially high in fibre and also contain vitamin E which is a very powerful antioxidant. Studies show they may even help reduce LDL (bad) cholesterol and insulin resistance which is common in those who are overweight.

Try to eat a range of nuts each day but not too many as they are high in good fat. These are some of the best to include in your diet: almonds, walnuts, pecans, cashews, Brazils, macadamias, pistachios and hazelnuts.

Super seeds

Seeds are a great source of protein, magnesium, zinc, calcium and omega 3 and 6 fatty acids. Pumpkin seeds, sesame seeds and sunflower seeds all make great snacks. However, they may not be suitable for young children who could choke.

Flax seed, chia seeds and linseed have all gained popularity recently and also offer the same health benefits as others. If flax seed has been properly processed then it will have a higher level of omega 3 and therefore offer greater health benefits especially in terms of heart health.

How can you combine seeds into your diet?

- Add them to bread you make or buy seeded loaves especially those with pumpkin and sunflower seeds
- Put a handful on your cereal - Especially with porridge, they add texture as well as flavour and nutrition
- Mix a handful into yoghurt or add to dried fruit
- Add to salads or other meals such as casseroles

Fill the gap

Leaving a long gap between meals allows your metabolism to slow down and therefore you burn calories slower too. Whilst the emphasis shouldn't just be on calorie burning, it is an essential part of weight loss in particular.

Eat at least three meals a day. Snacking is also ok too so long as it is healthy (see previous tips). It will keep your metabolism active. Leaving long gaps is also going to make you very hungry which is when you are most likely to start eating all the wrong foods and then eat a meal too.

If you are in a job which involves a lot of travel, try to take food with you in case you can't get anything nice to eat whilst you're on the road. For example, soup is great in a flask as it stays warm and won't go off quickly. Have some fruit, nuts and vegetable sticks already chopped up which you can easily snack on. Make a sandwich the night before and put it in a cool box so it doesn't get too warm. This is particularly important in summer but also if food is stored in the car and you have the heating on, it's more likely to go off.

Lovely lunches

Lunch seems to cause a lot of problems to a lot of people and there is no need for it to be that way, it just needs some planning and organisation.

If you have children and are making them a packed lunch, make yours at the same time. Making your own lunch not only saves you money but you also know what's gone into it and chances are it will be healthier.

Surprise children with adding a treat once or a twice a week but vary the days. This will keep them interested in packed lunches and encourage them to eat better.

Try different sandwich fillings and breads to make lunchtime more interesting. For example wraps, rolls and pitta breads make great alternatives to a sandwich. If you have cooked pasta or rice the night before you can also use that and make up a little salad for them and for you.

Soup is great during the winter time for adults and older children. If your workplace has a microwave you can also make meals such as egg or beans on toast and jacket potato with various fillings which will keep you going longer than a sandwich, packet of crisps or a chocolate bar.

What about fussy children and lunches?

Fussy children will eventually become less fussy although it may take years. When children are at school, it's much harder to regulate what they eat. Older children may be clever enough to throw food away that hasn't been eaten so you think they have finished their lunch.

If children have school lunches, it's also hard to monitor what they are eating. Whilst improvements have been made, there is a long way to go and children may just eat mash and gravy or something similar. If you have concerns, ask your school if they can monitor your child more closely.

You may find it easier to give your child a packed lunch.

Start with things they like and you know they might eat. Each week add a new food. Research suggests children need to try a food ten times before they either like or dislike it. If they haven't tried the food, sit down with them and try it with them. Even just putting it to their lips is a positive step. Do this with each new food and at dinner time too. It may take a while but will encourage children to try something new.

Delicious dinners

Do you make a different meal for every person in the household? Then stop! That's right, stop.

Making different meals is a waste of time, money and effort, all things we are short of these days. Ask yourself, 'why do I do it?' Then ask, 'do I really need to do it or is there another way?' Chances are there is an alternative and if that means somebody may have to have their dinner reheated later that's fine. So long as food is only reheated once after cooking it won't kill anyone. If it's because the children are fussy, read my next tip.

Cook one meal which can be easily portioned and reheated or put in the freezer for another day. Try to sit with your children when they eat even if you aren't eating and use it as a time to talk to them about their day. You will also establish better eating habits and table manners as you can guide them on what to do.

Top quick dinners:
- Stir fry with noodles and rice
- Spaghetti bolognaise
- Jacket potato with beans
- Homemade chicken nuggets and potato wedges with vegetables
- Sausage, mash and steamed vegetables

Tackling fussy eaters

I have already talked about fussy eaters but dinner time requires a different strategy as you are there with them.

Set out what you want them to eat/try when you all sit down. Make those expectations clear and then ignore the issue of food and talk to the child and others at the table about what everyone has done that day, the weather, what you're doing at the weekend. Anything that does not give that child more attention. More often than not children are craving the attention they get from being naughty and not eating, ignore it.

If you make meal times into a war zone, the situation becomes worse and there will be tears and tantrums which leave everyone unhappy. The child probably hasn't eaten anything and is hungry which is when they try to ask for other food they like. If this happens, you must not let them revert to favourites. They may be allowed something if they have eaten what you said at the table or you may choose to use something else as a treat.

Once you set out your expectations, stick to them and make sure you don't give in. This is difficult but if you do, the child will never have to do anything different as they know you don't mean what you say which will undermine you on every level.

Vile vegetables

How can you get children to eat vegetables when they don't like them? Hide them!

A lot of children hate vegetables and refuse to eat them which cause parents great concern but there are ways you can get children to eat them if you're a little bit cunning.

Chop vegetables finely and add them to sauces such as tomato. You can hide almost any vegetable in a tomato sauce with the exception of cauliflower and broccoli which don't work as well. Buy a blender so you can blitz sauces. Children will be none the wiser as to what's in them. Tomato sauce is great to have as a standby because you can make it into bolognaise, chilli or just add some pasta or rice with meatballs.

Try cooking them a different way. Roast vegetables are great for winter time and often vegetables taste sweeter when cooked that way especially parsnips and sweet potato. Some children prefer raw vegetables especially if you use them creatively e.g., to make funny faces on the plate. Try them with a dip such as humus for variety.

Five a day

It's a well-known fact that we need to eat five portions of fruit and vegetables daily but how do you manage it?

Children:
- Glass of orange or apple juice with breakfast
- Chopped banana or a handful of raisins on cereal
- Grapes for a mid-morning snack
- Carrot or cucumber sticks at lunch time
- Broccoli, baked beans, sweet corn, peas or cauliflower with dinner (include 2 if possible)

Adults:
- Glass of apple or orange juice with breakfast
- Chopped fruit on cereal
- Apple or pear for mid-morning snack
- Salad or a vegetable based soup for lunch or fruit as a dessert
- Banana for mid afternoon snack
- Vegetables with dinner

Try to include a variety of colours as this increases your intake of vitamins and minerals which are found in higher quantities in certain fruits and vegetables than others. Ordering a fruit and vegetable box can be a great way to encourage the whole family to try new foods and doesn't have to be expensive. If you have vegetables left over, cut them up, freeze them, then add to meals when required.

Why eat vegetables anyway?

Vegetables are full of vitamins and minerals plus fibre which our body needs for optimum health. The body needs fibre to help prevent constipation which can, in turn, lead to other bowel problems such as diverticular disease and possibly bowel cancer. Fibre adds the bulk to our poo which helps to excrete it from the body and increases transit time so waste does not sit inside you for too long. However, a very high fibre diet is ok for adults but can be too much for children, therefore they can't absorb all the nutrients they need.

We need vitamins and minerals to help boost our immune system and keep us generally healthy. Different coloured vegetables are rich in a variety of vitamins. For example the colour orange in carrots indicates they are high in beta carotene. Eating a rainbow of colours in your food will ensure you have an adequate intake of all the vitamins and minerals you need.

Vegetables also add bulk to your meals which help keep you feeling fuller for longer so you eat less later on. They should make up half of your plate at dinner. If you want to reduce carbohydrates, increase your vegetables as they are lower calorie alternatives.

Fabulous fruit

Fruit is often demonised because of its sugar content but it is actually a great source of vitamins and minerals like vegetables. Although fruit does contain sugar, it is natural sugar which is much less detrimental to health than processed sugar.

Citrus fruits such as oranges are high in vitamin C which boost your immune system and help fight coughs and colds. Other fruits contain fibre which is important for good digestive health (see previous tip) and all contain vitamins, minerals and antioxidants needed by the body for optimum condition.

Fruit makes a great snack and gives your body the nutrients it needs to cope with everyday life. We are exposed to pollutants (alcohol, cigarette smoke, chemicals in food, stress) and our body needs the vitamins and minerals in fruit to help keep us healthy. Antioxidants are particularly important for helping prevent diseases such as cancer, keeping our hearts healthy and reducing the risk of Alzheimer's because they scavenge the free radicals caused by the pollutants to which we are exposed.

Sugar - the demon?

Honestly, yes it is. Is it worse than fat? In most cases yes except for trans-fats, why? Mainly because it is so addictive but it's also less natural than some fats. The more sugar you consume, the more you want especially if it is refined like that used in chocolate, cakes, white bread etc. It has such a big impact on your blood sugar that once the body has processed it, it's desperate for more which can cause those mid-morning and afternoon sugar cravings.

So how do you deal with a sugar addiction?

Get rid of every low fat product in your house!

When fat is removed from food, sugar is added. Use full fat versions and just have a little less of it. Sugar is in almost everything that is processed whether it's sweet or savoury. You wouldn't put sugar in a lasagne if you made it at home but the food industry does.

Stop buying processed food and make your own. It sounds time consuming but if you are organised and batch cook, it doesn't need to be. Swap any white carbohydrates for wholemeal too. You will be doing wonders for your family's health by weaning them off so much sugar. Also, cut down sugar added to cereals and hot drinks. Do it a little bit at a time and no one will notice.

Carbohydrates - high GI v low GI?

The body needs carbohydrate despite what you may read.

As explained in the last tip, sugar is the bad form of it. It has the most effect on blood sugar and that's what we're trying to avoid as excess sugar is stored in the body as fat and the body releasing a lot of insulin to deal with excess sugar can also cause it to lay down fat. Most foods which are high in sugar (sweet foods) are high GI and these are the foods to cut down.

Carbohydrates such as wholemeal bread, pasta and brown rice plus potatoes and sweet potatoes have less of an effect on blood sugar and are also an important source of vitamins. These are known as low GI. For example, bread contains vitamin B and may be fortified with other minerals such as calcium and folic acid. Potatoes also contain vitamin C although only sweet potatoes count as a vegetable. They also have fibre in the skins which the body needs.

Consuming mainly low GI carbohydrates in appropriate portion sizes will not cause you to gain weight however, a large intake of high GI foods will as they generally don't leave you feeling very full causing you to snack more to satisfy cravings.

Low carbohydrate, high protein?

Eating a lower carbohydrate diet is ok for adults but not children who need a balanced diet to meet all their requirements. Try to give your child low GI carbohydrates where possible.

If you are going to reduce carbs, remove sugary snacks and cook evening meals which consist of more protein and vegetables such as fish and steamed veg or chicken and steamed veg/salad depending on the season. Low carbohydrate diets can be successful for weight loss because it is often carbohydrates to which people are addicted. White carbohydrates such as bread and pasta are particularly addictive. When carbohydrates are severely cut, the body can find it difficult at first and there may be side effects such as shaking, nausea and headaches but after a few days these will go as your body adjusts. Providing your intake of nutrients is sufficient, there is no reason why a healthy adult cannot follow a lower carbohydrate, higher protein diet.

Some people can exercise and follow a low carbohydrate diet but it takes some getting used to. If you are going to, make sure you first seek professional advice from a sports nutritionist or dietician.

Protein

Protein is essential in our diet to help build and repair muscle and grow.

In the UK, we are not protein deficient due to the high amount we consume but the type of protein you eat can have a big impact on your body.

Choose lean protein sources such as meat and fish to help the whole family grow fit and strong. Although bacon, sausages and burgers do contain meat, their percentage is often lower and they may be high in salt or have other ingredients such as rusk added. Try to buy these from a reputable butcher where the meat content will be higher and eat no more than once a week. Avoid highly processed burgers and hot dogs.

Pulses such as kidney beans, butter beans, cannellini beans and haricot beans all provide protein too. Legumes are also a great source of protein for example lentils and quinoa are now hugely popular and while having a high protein content they also have a starchier taste and appearance. Add them to meals such as stews and casseroles, sauces and soups and you will be increasing the protein and fibre content.

Legumes- friend or foe?

Start eating legumes once a week or more. They are a great addition to any diet whether you're vegetarian or not. If you are vegetarian, they should make up a large percentage of your food intake due to the protein they contain.

Most of us eat baked beans on a fairly regular basis and whilst being a little higher in sugar and salt, they are essentially healthy. Start adding them to your family's meals to increase the fibre content. The UK does not consume enough fibre, pulses and lentils are a fantastic source. They are also incredibly cheap and can add bulk to other dishes which may mean you can use less meat which is much more expensive.

You can use legumes in:

- Casseroles
- Soups - lentils can thicken soup
- Chilli - reduce the meat content and add some pulses
- Your own baked beans
- Salads - 3 bean salad
- Homemade vegetarian burgers
- Mash - use butterbeans instead of potatoes

Help! My child wants to be vegetarian!

It's very common for children to go through phases of wanting to be vegetarian or refusing to eat certain foods. Unless you are strongly against it or it is going to be bad for their health, such as cutting out food groups, let them try it. Serve them a completely vegetarian meal and see what they think. Most children don't particularly like it and revert to eating meat and fish

You could compromise and do some vegetarian meals and some meat or fish meals but explain your expectations at each meal to ensure they eat enough and it's not just carbohydrates and vegetables they're eating.

Include plenty of pulses or lentils in vegetarian meals to help fill your child up so they are less likely to snack between meals due to hunger. A vegetarian diet can be very healthy but there is a tendency to consume excessive amounts of cheese as it is more filling and also snacking on junk such as crisps and chocolate. If your child is hungry, encourage them to snack on fruit, nuts or vegetable sticks with a dip such as humus which is slightly healthier than others available on the market.

Fabulous fish

In the UK, we vastly underrate fish. It is fantastic! Not just oily fish but all kinds of fish. Include it in your diet at least once if not twice a week. Pregnant women should only consume oily fish once a week and avoid those with higher mercury content such as shark, tuna and swordfish (plus others).

Fish is a fantastic source of lean protein and a great alternative to meat especially for vegetarians (some eat fish but not meat depending on type) who won't eat meat but will eat fish. It is also very quick to cook and versatile. You can make it spicy, plain, add a sauce, bake it in the oven in a parcel, grill it, fry it or make it into a stew.

Try some less commonly eaten fish such as cuttlefish which is relatively cheap, has a more meaty flavour and works well in a stew. If your family do not like fish, choose a more meaty variety which has a less strong fish flavour. If you buy from a fishmonger, you can ask them to de-bone the fish and remove the skin and head plus anything else you think might put people off eating it.

Oily fish

Oily fish has numerous health advantages but we do not eat enough of it to gain those benefits from the omega 3's found in it. So why is omega 3 important?

There have been numerous studies suggesting a range of benefits of consuming omega 3 but the most conclusive evidence is around asthma and allergy in childhood, heart diseases (lowers cholesterol), cancer and possible protection against cognitive decline in later years.

Omega 3 thins the blood making it less likely to clot which is a major cause of heart attack. By lowering LDL (bad) cholesterol, there is less plaque build-up in the arteries allowing blood to flow through more easily. Blood is also less sticky.

Fish oil supplements have been shown to have no real benefit to health, better to eat oily fish for omega 3.

Which fish are oily?
- Fresh tuna (not canned)
- Fresh and tinned salmon
- Mackerel
- Trout
- Sardines
- Pilchards
- Herring
- Kippers
- Whitebait
- Eel

I don't like fish but want to increase my omega 3 intake

There are also plant sources of omega 3 which should be included in the diet whether you are vegetarian or not.

Omega 3 can be found in properly processed flax seed, hulled hempseed, chia seeds, rapeseed oil and walnuts. Try to include one of these in your diet each day for optimum health.

Stir a spoonful of flax, hemp or chia seeds into your porridge in the morning or add to cereals. Chia seeds are commonly eaten by themselves and other seeds can be added to a fruit, nut and seed medley which makes a great snack. You could make your own bread including seeds to give a more interesting flavour, texture and a host of health benefits for the whole family.

Rapeseed oil can be used for cooking although some of its properties may be lost at higher temperatures. For frying, use good quality olive oil. Rapeseed oil can be used for dressings and as an alternative to butter in some cakes.

Fat - will it make me fat?

The answer is not necessarily. We all need fat because it is a source of important vitamins. Vitamin A is found in fat, some foods contain small amounts of vitamin D and others contain vitamin E. Just as we need the vitamins from fruit and vegetables, we need the vitamins from fat.

An excessive consumption of anything will have negative effects on your body and yes, eating too much fat will make you fat but equally eating too much sugar will make you fat. However, fat is more satiating than carbohydrate and so will keep you feeling fuller for longer meaning you eat less over the course of a day. Choose lean sources such as unprocessed meat and fish.

Fat also has health properties and our bodies need it to stay healthy, keep us warm and protect our vital organs. Our bodies need the essential fatty acids and also monounsaturated fats (the cis form not trans form) and polyunsaturated fatty acids.

Including a wide range of foods in your diet will ensure you eat a variety of the different types of fat. Trans-fats are usually found in processed food but their usage has decreased considerably over the past few years.

The not so nice fats

There are some fats which are not so nice - hydrogenated fats. These are the ones we should be limiting in our diets. They are mainly found in processed food so again, the more real food you eat, the less likely you are to be consuming high amounts of these.

Eat food in its true state and again avoid the low fat options as these are often filled with artificial ingredients to make them taste nice, look nice, last longer and replicate the full fat versions.

Did you know that by law, margarine must contain the same fat content as butter? You are better off eating butter which is less processed and has much fewer artificial ingredients than margarine.

What about saturated fats? Saturated fats are much disputed and confusing evidence can be found for them harming health but also that they do no harm.

Eat food in its state closest to nature. For example a piece of steak which has been grilled may contain saturated fat but most of the fat drains out of the meat during cooking especially if it is grilled or baked on a rack and it has not had any fat added to it. Everything in moderation is the key.

Salt

We are constantly told we need to reduce our salt intake but how?

First, stop adding it to food at the table and in cooking!

Second, once again, stop buying processed food. There is a lot of hidden salt in bread so make your own. Sounds time consuming? Buy a bread maker (they're not expensive) and you can add your own ingredients and monitor how much salt you use. It takes five minutes to put all the ingredients in and then you can leave it to sort itself out.

Swap cereal for porridge or muesli which generally doesn't have salt added. Look at the labels to see how much salt is in a product and go for something with less than 0.3g of salt per 100g or 120mg sodium.

Remember though, we do need some salt in our diet so don't cut it out completely. We should eat around 6g a day which is the equivalent of a teaspoon. If you exercise and sweat heavily, you may need to add a little salt to your diet depending on what you're doing but for the average person, you don't.

Ready meals

Remove the ready meals! Ready meals are a huge waste of money. They contain very little nutritional value and generally taste pretty disgusting with the exception of a few from the high end supermarkets which are expensive.

The meat and vegetable content of ready meals is generally low and they are full of artificial ingredients, added sugar, salt and fat. Very few contribute to your 5 a day and most contain ingredients you would never put in meals at home.

If you are looking to lose weight, ready meals are a definite no as they are small portions, high in fat and sugar but don't keep you feeling very full for long.

Stop feeding them to your children and family!! In the next tip I show you how to make your own in no time at all.

Cooking meals from scratch is not difficult, expensive or time consuming but while you may need to be a little more organised the benefits are huge. I talk more about that later on in the book.

Make your own ready meals - really?

Yes really. Make your own ready meals and put them in the freezer so all you have to do is defrost, reheat and add vegetables. How easy is that?

Batch cook your meals so if you make a bolognaise sauce, make double the amount and then portion it up and freeze it. Your own ready meals are much healthier than anything you will buy in the supermarket and much cheaper. Most meals will freeze and defrost really well.

Buy some foil trays, the ones with the cardboard lids are great and you can easily write on them so you know what you have; include the date of freezing.

Having ready meals in the freezer will also make sure you don't need takeaways or that you have to rely on dinner being beans on toast again because there is nothing else in the house.

This is key to helping your whole family eat well, stay healthy and if necessary lose weight. However, a good habit to adopt in general is to ensure that whatever is frozen is defrosted before cooking.

Super slow cookers

Go and buy a slow cooker! They are usually not expensive but will transform your life and the food you eat.

Slow cookers make home cooking so easy and healthy. You can cook almost anything in one - casseroles, chilli, curry - anything. If you are working, prepare the ingredients the night before and store it in the fridge, the meat may need to be browned first. You can then throw everything in the slow cooker in the morning and switch it on as you walk out of the door. When you walk in, dinner is ready and may only need some carbohydrates and fresh vegetables to go with it.

Most recipes suitable for a slow cooker can be frozen too which creates your home made ready meals. Slow cooked meals are really nutritious if you put vegetables in too because all the vitamins that leach out, end up in the gravy/sauce of the meal.

Sweet: savoury

As a nation, we consume far too much sugar and need to cut it down.

Think about how much sugar do you and your family eat at the moment? Think about all that hidden sugar that you're probably consuming too. Is it frightening? Probably.

So, look at the ratio of sweet to savoury food in your diet. You should be eating much more savoury food such as meat, fish, rice, potatoes, vegetables and less of the sweet such as cakes, biscuits, chocolate etc. If you do have to have some sweet foods minimise it, aim for a ratio of 2 savoury to 1 sweet.

Sweet food is generally what is addictive, has no nutritional value but a lot of calories and may be the reason you have gained weight, feel tired and lethargic and often not feeling at your best. There is also junk savoury food of course such as crisps, sausage rolls, pork pies etc., be mindful of what you eat and how much of it you consume. Again, preparing some carrot sticks and eating those with a healthy dip will make you feel much better than eating an ice-cream or packet of crisps.

Cut the comfort eating

This is a very common issue which men, women and a rising number of children have adopted.

Comfort eating is something which can only be tackled when the time is right. It is generally fuelled by unhappiness caused by something in your life be it worry, stress, money issues, relationship issues, job issues or ironically malnutrition from comfort eating.

Sometimes we eat out of boredom. Ask yourself if you are really hungry and are you going to feel better from eating junk? If the answer is no and you know it will make you feel worse, try to find something else to do. Do something positive that will take your mind off food. Go for a walk, swim or stroll in the garden. If it's at night, read a book or do an exercise DVD to focus your mind on the positives of being healthy. Stop eating food whilst you're watching TV, that's just bad on so many levels.

If it's a child who is sneaking food, try and talk to them but you may need to avoid the direct subject but instead ask about them and their day. As they talk, you may pick up reasons which could cause comfort eating. Discuss a strategy with them and strive to have less junk food available in the house. You might ask them to help you to create better meals; children often love to learn how to cook and sometimes asking children to teach us empowers them (and us) to learn more.

Eat as a family

If you want your children to develop good eating habits, they need to see you eat. Children learn behaviours and copy from others.

It's not always possible to sit down and eat together but that should be the goal, make an effort to eat with your children as much as you can. Even if it's only possible for someone to sit with them at breakfast, they will see you eat a healthy meal and understand that they should too. Try to eat fruit or vegetables in front of them and encourage them to try new foods with you. If they see you eat vegetables with your meal, it will become more of a habit for them and they assume it's the norm. Try to eat with children from when they are just weaning to establish good habits from a young age.

When you all eat together, children will also learn table manners and social skills and it is an opportunity for you all to sit down and talk as a family.

If you have fussy eaters (see my fussy eating tips) ignore bad behaviour at the table and set expectations.

Consider making meal-times less about the food and more about social interaction.

Planning is key

As they say, when you fail to plan, you plan to fail. Make a meal plan each week and write a shopping list to go with it or obtain one from my website. If you don't have a plan, you won't have the right ingredients in the cupboard to make a meal and you will be more likely to resort to ready meals, takeaways or other unhealthy options for dinner.

Writing a meal plan will only take a few minutes but will save last minute supermarket trips and also saves food waste. You buy the amount of food you need for the week, possibly extra to batch cook meals and you won't need to worry about it for another week.

Money is tight for a lot of people and throwing out food is just like throwing away money. Also making too many trips to the shops costs you more in time and money so planning to buy well will help you save and give you more hours back to use elsewhere.

Buy the amount of food you need and freeze leftovers rather than be tempted to serve up bigger portions or give/eat seconds.

If you are losing weight, planning is even more important as it helps stop mindless eating and snacking because when there is nothing in the house to eat you risk either not bothering or you exist on toast.

What about if we have visitors?

Having visitors is not an excuse for all your good habits to go out the window. Your visitors should, within reason, eat what you put in front of them and therefore you can put healthy food on the table.

There's no need to buy huge amounts of food like crisps and dips for them as people generally don't need them. Do your guests a favour and look after their waistlines as well as your own!

Depending on the people visiting, you may consume more alcohol than normal. You can either choose to accept this and view it as a treat weekend or drink less and be more restrained. If you have visitors regularly, drinking less may be the better option otherwise the alcohol intake increases significantly at the weekend.

If close friends you may wish to confide to your visitors that you are losing weight and you would welcome their support.

Definitely do not provide junk food and expect others to avoid it just because you are making that lifestyle choice. If you provide snacks to eat make them healthier ones and you may well find that your guests will appreciate the effort you have taken, after all, anyone can tip crisps into a bowl.

If being healthier is your goal, you may choose to indulge a little as a treat and go back to healthy eating afterwards.

What if we're going away?

Going away to a friends and family and going away on holiday are two different situations.

If you're going to friends and family, you may want to explain you're losing weight or just enjoy the time you are away. If you choose to indulge, be sensible and take small amounts. Although you don't have much control at other people's homes, it can be easier to say no or take small amounts. You can also do more exercise such as suggesting a walk after lunch.

Going on holiday can be much harder. However, it doesn't mean you can't still keep up good habits. Most people drink and eat more on holiday but you can make some clever choices. Firstly, if it's hot, you need to make sure you're drinking plenty of water, even more if you're drinking alcohol too. Alternate alcoholic and non-alcoholic drinks.

Secondly, make wise choices about what you eat (see next tip). If it's very hot, you might not feel like as much to eat and you may lean towards lighter meals such as salad anyway.

Try to do some exercise. Go swimming every day if there is a pool nearby or walk to places or along the beach.

Eating out

There's no reason why eating out has to equal loads of calories and feeling so full you can't move if you make some sensible choices.

When you're eating out, choose sauces which aren't cream based and remember you can always leave things like the chips and just eat the protein and vegetables. Ask for something as a starter sized portion or simply choose to have a starter as a main course. If you are choosing salad, ask for it without the dressing as that can make a salad highly calorific.

If you are a desert person, why not have a starter and desert? There's no need to eat three courses for the sake of it. If you are desperate to have desert consider sharing with a companion.

Set yourself a rule before you go and stick to it. If you find it hard not to over indulge, tell a friend or your partner that you don't want to have three courses and not to let you have them. Remember alcohol has a lot of calories so drinking less will make a night out less calorific meaning you have less to burn off.

Excellent exercise

Exercise has so many benefits for the whole family but is often pushed way down the priority list. Push exercise up the list and make time for it! Schedule it into your diary and do it. No excuses, you need to exercise.

Exercise doesn't have to be three hours in the gym it can be a walk or cycle ride. Gardening and cleaning are both good forms of exercise and may suit older people who don't like the idea of a gym. Try cleaning the car yourself rather than taking it to a car wash. Whatever form it takes aim for 30 minutes 5 times a week.

If you struggle to build exercise into your routine:

- Get off the bus a stop earlier
- Cycle or walk to work/school
- Do an exercise DVD once the children are in bed
- Find a buddy and go running
- Use stairs instead of an elevator
- Park further away at shops, work or the gym so you walk more

Exercise not only has benefits for your physical health because it helps with weight loss, blood pressure control, heart health and respiratory function. It also has benefits for your mental health, in particular, depression and anxiety.

Family friendly exercise

Children need exercise too. They might run around like mad things but they also need to go outside and exercise. Lots of sports centres offer classes for pre-school children such as dancing, gymnastics etc., and it's important to take them to try them if you can.

Exercise is important for helping to keep children active and will also help them develop muscle and peak bone mass. The higher peak bone mass, the less likely they are to develop osteoporosis later in life.

Do something as a family. Go to the park after school or at the weekend. It's free and children love it. Take a football or their bikes and let them burn off steam. A family bike ride can be great especially if you have nice cycle paths near you which are away from cars and much safer for young children. Even playing football in the garden is a great form of exercise.

Most children love swimming and taking them from a young age will help get over any fears they may have. Go regularly if you can so they keep up their confidence.

Keep a diary

Just like you might keep a diet diary, keep an exercise diary and write down what you did and how much you achieved each time you exercise. You will be amazed how quickly your fitness improves and how motivating it is to see that improvement.

Write down the exercise you do, how long for, the intensity and how you feel. Each week you will notice you can exercise for longer and find it easier. Be prepared, there may be weeks when that doesn't happen especially if you have been ill.

You may also find it useful to write down any observations around what you have eaten and how you perform. It can be motivating to look back and see your progress especially on the odd occasion when you may feel like you are struggling. Everyone goes through some barriers but the important thing is to work past those, when you do you will soon feel on top form again.

Have a goal in mind. It might be you want to build up to run 5k, you might set a target to be able to cover that distance at the end of say 3 months initially. Once you have reached your goal, set another to give you something to focus on and train towards.

Refer to your diary often and very quickly you will recognise the positive changes that you have made.

Exercise at work?

Really? Can you really exercise at work? Yes!

If you catch a train or bus to work get off a stop earlier and walk; you will also save money on the fare.

If you drive to work can you park farther away and walk the extra distance?

If you have a lift in your building, stop using it and start taking the stairs. Even if you work several flights up, get out of the lift before your floor and walk up increasing the distance each week. You can also walk a lot further down stairs because it takes less effort so start doing that. You may also find that its quicker so you'll get some more minutes back into your day.

If you work at a desk get up regularly and walk the long way around to get a drink or go to the bathroom. Go for a walk in your lunch break and encourage others to join you. Get the whole workplace healthier and it will be a more productive environment.

When you're sitting at your desk, do leg raises under the desk. Just lift your legs together and then lower them and repeat so you work your abs. Gradually build up the amount you do and hold them for longer to improve muscle tone.

Live your life!

Whilst what you eat, drink and the amount of exercise you do has a huge impact on your existence, you only get one life and it's important not to become so bogged down with trying to be healthy the whole time that it becomes an obsession.

Eating disorders are on the rise in both men and women and more worryingly in children from a much younger age than previously seen. This is partly down to our obsession with weight, size and looks along with availability of fast, processed foods.

Remember, being healthy is much more important than being skinny. Have a little bit of what you fancy and bear in mind the saying 'everything in moderation'.

Eat a mostly healthy diet but accept that it is ok to enjoy a treat every now and then. Strong not stick thin is far healthier.

Food should be healthy and enjoyable but it should not be the main focus of your attention. So, as you adopt and maintain a healthy diet, start to enjoy all aspects of your life and look forward to it being longer and happier.

Adopting a positive attitude to what you consume may well be the inspiration you need to be the person you strive to be.

Appendix

Adams et al., 2010. Lifestyle factors and ghrelin: critical review and implications for weight loss maintenance. [online]. *Obesity Reviews*. 12, **5**, pp 211-218. Last accessed on 21.1.13 at: www.onlinelibrary.wiley.com/doi/10.1111/j.1467-789X.2010.00776.x/pdf

Chaphut et al., 2011. The Association Between Short Sleep Duration and Weight Gain is Dependent on Disinhibited Eating Behaviour in Adults. [online]. *Sleep*. 34, **10**, pp.1291-1297. Last accessed on 21.1.13 at: www.ncbi.nlm.nih.gov/pmc/articles/PMC3174831/

Yang, Q., 2010. Gain weight by "going diet?" Artificial sweeteners and the neurobiology of sugar cravings. [online]. *Yale Journal of Biology and Medicine*. 83, **2**, pp. 101-108. Last accessed on 21.1.13 at: www.ncbi.nlm.nih.gov/pmc/articles/PMC2892765/

Van der Heijden et al., 2012. A Prospective Study of Breakfast Consumption and Weight Gain Among US Men. [online]. *Obesity*. 15, **10**, pp. 2463-2469. Last accessed on 21.1.13 at: www.onlinelibrary.wiley.com/doi/10.1038/oby.2007.292/pdf

Vinson. J. A. and Cai. Y., 2011. Nuts, especially walnuts, have both antioxidant quantity and efficacy and exhibit significant potential health benefits. [online]. *Food Functions*. 3, pp. 134-140. Last accessed on 21.1.13 at: www.pubs.rsc.org/en/content/articlepdf/2012/FO/C2FO10152A

Kendall *et al.,* 2010. Health benefits of nuts in prevention and management of diabetes. [online]. *Asia Pacific Journal of Clinical Nutrition.* 19, **1**, pp. 110-116. Last accessed on 21.1.13 at:
www.211.76.170.15/server/APJCN/Volume19/vol19.1/Finished/15_1734_110-116.pdf

Anderson *et al.,* 2009. Health benefits of dietary fiber. [online]. *Nutrition Reviews.* 67, **4**, pp. 188-205. Last accessed on 21.1.13 at:
www.onlinelibrary.wiley.com/doi/10.1111/j.1753-4887.2009.00189.x/pdf

Dias. J. S., 2012. Nutritional Quality and Health Benefits of Vegetables: A Review. [online]. *Scientific Research.* 3, **10**, pp. 1354-1374. Last accessed on 21.1.13 at:
www.scirp.org/journal/PaperInformation.aspx?PaperID=23384

Larsen *et al.,* 2010. Diets with High or Low Protein Content and Glycaemic Index for Weight-Loss Maintenance. [online]. *The New England Journal of Medicine.* 363. Pp. 2102-2113. Last accessed on 21.1.13 at:
www.nejm.org/doi/pdf/10.1056/NEJMoa1007137

Wylie- Rosett *et al.,* 2012. Carbohydrates and Increases in Obesity: Does the Type of Carbohydrate Make a Difference? [online]. *Obesity Research.* 12, **11**, pp. 124-129. Last accessed on 21.1.13 at:
www.onlinelibrary.wiley.com/doi/10.1038/oby.2004.277/pdf

Welch *et al.*, 2010. Dietary intake and status of n-3 polyunsaturated fatty acids in a population of fish-eating and non-fish-eating meat eaters, vegetarians and vegans and the precursor product ratio of a-linolenic acid to long-chain n-3 polyunsaturated fatty acids: results from the EPIC-Norfolk cohort. [online]. *The American Journal of Clinical Nutrition.* 92, **5**, pp. 1040-1051. Last accessed on 21.1.13 at: www.ajcn.nutrition.org/content/92/5/1040.full.pdf+html

Roos *et al.*, 2012. Fish as a dietary source of healthy long chain n-3 polyunsaturated fatty acids (LC n-3 PUFA) and vitamin D: A Review of Current Literature. [online]. *The Food and Health Innovation Service.* Last accessed on 21.1.13 at: www.foodhealthinnovation.com/media/5756/fish_final_june_201 2.pdf